About the NCCN Guidelines for Patients®

NCCN National Comprehensive Cancer Network®

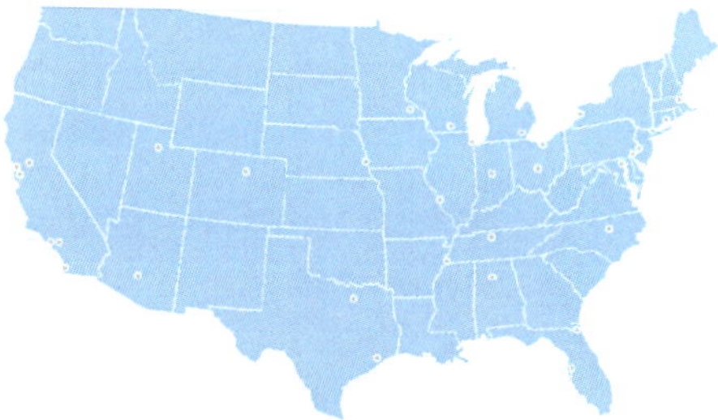

Did you know that top cancer centers across the United States work together to improve cancer care? This alliance of leading cancer centers is called the National Comprehensive Cancer Network® (NCCN®).

Cancer care is always changing. NCCN develops evidence-based cancer care recommendations used by health care providers worldwide. These frequently updated recommendations are the NCCN Clinical Practice Guidelines in Oncology (NCCN Guidelines®). The NCCN Guidelines for Patients plainly explain these expert recommendations for people with cancer and caregivers.

These NCCN Guidelines for Patients are based on the NCCN Clinical Practice Guidelines in Oncology (NCCN Guidelines®) for Palliative Care Version 2.2023 – April 24, 2023.

View the NCCN Guidelines for Patients free online
NCCN.org/patientguidelines

Find an NCCN Cancer Center near you
NCCN.org/cancercenters

Connect with us

Supporters

NCCN Guidelines for Patients are supported by funding from the NCCN Foundation®

NCCN Foundation gratefully acknowledges the following corporate supporters for helping to make available these NCCN Guidelines for Patients: AstraZeneca, Baxter International Inc., Exelixis, GSK, Ipsen Biopharmaceuticals, Inc., and Karyopharm Therapeutics.

NCCN independently adapts, updates, and hosts the NCCN Guidelines for Patients. Our corporate supporters do not participate in the development of the NCCN Guidelines for Patients and are not responsible for the content and recommendations contained therein.

To make a gift or learn more, visit online or email

NCCNFoundation.org/donate

PatientGuidelines@NCCN.org

Contents

4 About palliative care

9 Managing distressing symptoms

18 Communicating with your care team

23 Making treatment decisions

34 Words to know

36 NCCN Contributors

37 NCCN Cancer Centers

40 Index

NCCN Foundation seeks to support the millions of patients and their families affected by a cancer diagnosis by funding and distributing NCCN Guidelines for Patients. NCCN Foundation is also committed to advancing cancer treatment by funding the nation's promising doctors at the center of innovation in cancer research. For more details and the full library of patient and caregiver resources, visit NCCN.org/patients.

National Comprehensive Cancer Network (NCCN) and NCCN Foundation
3025 Chemical Road, Suite 100, Plymouth Meeting, PA 19462 USA

1

About palliative care

5 What is palliative care?

5 Cancer care team

7 Palliative care specialists

8 Key points

Palliative care is an approach to health care for people living with serious illnesses, including cancer. It focuses on providing relief from the symptoms and stress of having cancer. The goal is to improve quality of life for both the person with cancer and their family and/or caregivers.

What is palliative care?

Palliative care is an important part of high-quality, comprehensive cancer care. The goal of palliative care is to control symptoms, relieve emotional and physical suffering that comes from the diagnosis and treatment of cancer, and improve quality of life for those with cancer and their families and/or caregivers. It is appropriate for anyone, regardless of age, cancer stage, or the need for other therapies.

How does palliative care fit into my cancer care?

Palliative care is part of your cancer care. It can begin at the time of diagnosis, be given during cancer treatment, and continue after treatment is complete.

Palliative care aims to help those with cancer:

- Control pain and other symptoms
- Manage distress
- Gain an understanding of the nature of the illness and what to expect in the future
- Have a sense of control over their disease and decisions
- Understand their illness and evaluate treatment options that align with their values and beliefs
- Discuss advance care planning
- Name decision makers in case of loss of decision-making ability
- Feel supported and provide an extra layer of support
- Ease burden on family members and strengthen relationships

Cancer care team

Treating cancer takes a team of people from different professional backgrounds who have knowledge (expertise) and experience in your type of cancer. Some members of your care team will be with you throughout cancer treatment, while others will only be there for parts of it.

Depending on your diagnosis, your team might include the following:

- **Oncologists** specialize in diagnosing and treating cancer. Types of oncologists include medical, radiation, and surgical oncologists.
- **Palliative care specialists** specialize in putting you at the center of your care and concentrate on preventing and alleviating suffering and improving quality of life.
- **Oncology nurses** provide your hands-on care, like giving systemic therapy, managing your care, answering questions, and helping you cope with side effects.
- **Oncology pharmacists** are experts in knowing how to use medicines to treat cancer and to manage symptoms and side effects.
- **Radiation therapists** provide your hands-on delivery of radiotherapy treatments.
- **Nutritionists and dietitians** can provide guidance on what foods are most suitable for your condition.
- **An occupational therapist** helps people with the tasks of daily living.
- **A physical therapist** helps people move with greater comfort and ease.
- **A certified lymphedema therapist** gives a type of massage called manual lymph drainage.
- **Psychologists and psychiatrists** are mental health experts who can help manage issues such as depression, anxiety, or other mental health conditions that can affect how you think, behave, and feel.
- **Social workers** help people solve and cope with problems in their everyday lives. Clinical social workers also diagnose and treat mental, behavioral, and emotional conditions. They, or other designated professionals, can help navigate the complexities of financial and insurance stresses.
- **Spiritual care specialists** identify and support those with spiritual distress or unmet spiritual needs.

What's the difference between palliative care and hospice?

Hospice care is specifically designed for individuals with a limited life expectancy. It focuses on providing comfort and support to people and their families by providing care providers and resources that specialize in end-of-life (EOL) care.

Palliative care specialists

Palliative care specialists work as part of a team that may include doctors, nurses, social workers, chaplains, and pharmacists. It may also include registered dieticians, occupational therapists, physical therapists, and psychologists. Palliative care specialists provide an extra layer of support and can be found in hospitals, outpatient centers, or in the community.

The palliative care team works together with you and your other health care providers to ensure you are at the center of conversations and decision-making about your cancer care.

The palliative care team may provide:

- Expert management of complex physical and emotional symptoms, including pain, depression, anxiety, fatigue, shortness of breath, constipation, nausea, loss of appetite, and difficulty sleeping
- Time to devote to family meetings and patient/family counseling
- Skilled communication about what to expect in the future in order to ensure that care is matched to the goals and priorities of the person with cancer and their family
- Coordination and communication of care plans among all health care providers and across all settings

When is palliative care given?

Palliative care is appropriate for any cancer stage and any cancer diagnosis.

Palliative care aims to:

- ✓ Manage symptoms and relieve suffering in all stages of disease, regardless of prognosis
- ✓ Align with your preferences and values
- ✓ Offer psychosocial, spiritual, and practical support for both you and your family and/or caregivers
- ✓ Coordinate and communicate with all those involved in your care

Palliative care teams may also be involved in the care of children and teens, whether they have cancer or are the children of adults with cancer. Because of the unique needs in this group, a palliative care team may include additional specialists such as those who work in child life services. Child life services help children cope with the stress and fear of being in a hospital.

Key points

- Palliative care is an approach to health care for people living with serious illnesses, including cancer.
- The goal of palliative care is to control symptoms, relieve emotional and physical suffering that comes from the diagnosis and treatment of cancer, and improve quality of life for those with cancer and their families and/or caregivers.
- Your palliative care team works together with you and your other health care providers to ensure you are at the center of conversations and decision-making about your cancer care.

2
Managing distressing symptoms

10 Physical symptoms

14 Psychosocial and spiritual distress

17 Key points

This chapter describes an overview of general symptoms and emotional, social, and spiritual needs that might affect quality of life. Your well-being is important. Share with your care team how you are feeling.

Physical symptoms

Physical symptoms may be uncomfortable and distressing. Share with your care team any concerns you may have. It is important to voice how you are feeling and any changes you have noticed so you can get the treatment you need.

The following pages discuss general situations and symptoms that might suggest the need for palliative care involvement. Pain and difficulty breathing are common physical symptoms experienced by those with cancer.

What's the difference between a sign and symptom?

A sign can be seen by someone else like your health care provider (HCP). A symptom is something only you can feel. It is important to tell your HCP if something doesn't feel or look right. Don't wait to say something!

You might be asked to describe your symptoms, their frequency, and how much they bother (distress) you. Your care team will try to anticipate symptoms, discuss how to prevent symptoms, and explain what to do if you have certain symptoms. Many cancer symptoms can be relieved with cancer treatment. Cancer treatment aims to control, or kill, cancer cells. Other symptoms can be treated with medicine or non-medicine treatments.

Constipation

In constipation, stool (poop) is hard, dry, and difficult to pass, and bowel movements don't happen very often. Other symptoms may include painful bowel movements, and feeling bloated, uncomfortable, and sluggish. Constipation is common in those who are treated with opioids. Other medicines and some cancers can cause constipation. In addition to physical discomfort, constipation can cause distress and anxiety. Medicine may be given to prevent or manage constipation.

Delirium

Delirium is a mental state in which you are confused, disoriented, and not able to think or remember clearly. It is a fast-developing type of confusion that makes it hard to concentrate or stay alert. It happens when your brain is not working as it should for various reasons. People with delirium often act very differently from their usual selves.

The following may help reduce delirium:

- Controlling the environment, which includes making sure that the room is quiet, calm, and well-lit; having clocks or calendars in view; and having family members around.
- Reducing or changing medicines that might be causing delirium.

- If needed, making sure that the person has a hearing aid, glasses, or other devices for communication

Diarrhea

Diarrhea is frequent and watery bowel movements, or more bowel movements than usual. It is a common side effect of chemotherapy. The severity (grade) and cause of diarrhea might be rated using a scoring system. Diarrhea is treated with prescription and over-the-counter (OTC) medicines, and food recommendations (like eating rice or bread). Avoid taking OTC medicines without speaking to your care team first. It is possible for diarrhea medicines to cause constipation or have other side effects. Ask your care team how to manage diarrhea and constipation.

Difficulty breathing

Difficulty breathing or shortness of breath (called dyspnea) is a very common symptom. How it feels and the level of discomfort is different for everyone. Non-medicine therapies are recommended such as the use of handheld fans directed at the face, cooler temperatures, stress management, relaxation therapy, and emotional and psychosocial support. Depending on the cause or the type of discomfort, medicine or other treatments might be given.

Supportive care resources

More information on supportive care is available at: NCCN.org/patientguidelines and on the NCCN Patient Guides for Cancer app.

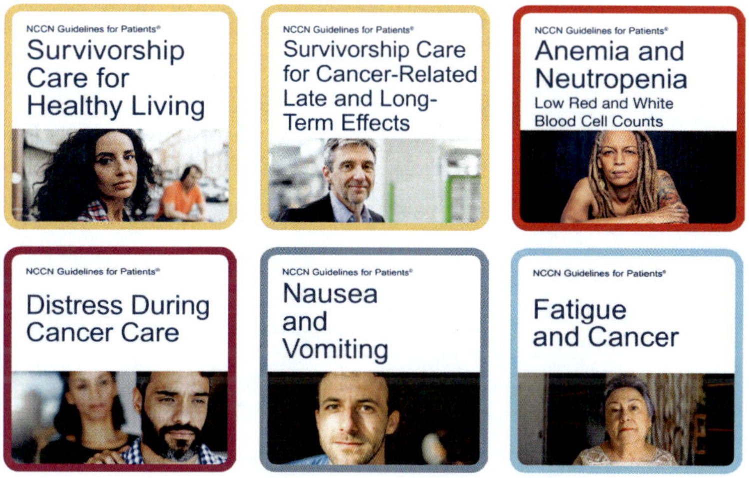

Difficulty eating

Many with cancer lose the desire to eat (anorexia) and don't feel hungry. Treatment or cancer can cause nausea and vomiting, mouth sores, food to taste differently, digestion issues, and pain. Your care team will look at the rate and severity of weight loss, if there is difficulty eating or digesting, and what might be causing the weight loss, among other things. You might have a swallowing evaluation. If you are having difficulty with eating, your team may ask you to meet with a registered dietitian, who is an expert in nutrition and food. Speak to your care team if you have trouble eating or maintaining weight.

Fatigue

Fatigue is extreme tiredness and inability to function due to lack of energy. Fatigue may be caused by cancer or it may be a side effect of treatment. Let your care team know how you are feeling and if fatigue is getting in the way of doing the things you enjoy. Eating a balanced diet, exercise, yoga, acupuncture, and massage therapy may help. You might be referred to a nutritionist or dietitian to help with fatigue.

For more information, see NCCN Guidelines for Patients: Fatigue and Cancer, available at NCCN.org/patientguidelines and on the NCCN Patient Guides for Cancer app.

Lymphedema

Lymphedema is a condition in which extra lymph fluid builds up in tissues and causes swelling. It may be caused when part of the lymph system is damaged or blocked, such as from surgery to remove lymph nodes or from radiation therapy. Cancers that block lymph vessels can also cause lymphedema. Swelling usually develops slowly over time. It may develop during treatment or it may start years after treatment. If you have lymphedema, you may be referred to an expert in lymphedema management. The swelling may be reduced by exercise, massage, compression sleeves, and other means.

For more information, see NCCN Guidelines for Patients: Survivorship Care for Cancer-Related Late and Long-Term Effects, available at NCCN.org/patientguidelines and on the NCCN Patient Guides for Cancer app.

Nausea and vomiting

Nausea and vomiting can be caused by cancer or its treatment. There are many medicines available to prevent nausea and vomiting. Often, these medicines work very well. One cause of nausea and vomiting might be a tumor blocking part of the bowel. Call your care team if you have nausea and vomiting that is new or worsening.

For more information, see NCCN Guidelines for Patients: Nausea and Vomiting available at NCCN.org/patientguidelines and on the NCCN Patient Guides for Cancer app.

Pain

Pain is an unpleasant sensory and emotional experience. Pain can be caused by cancer or cancer treatment. Controlling symptoms and managing pain is an important part of cancer care.

Pain is a very subjective experience. Everyone feels pain differently. Some people are very sensitive to pain. Some people can tolerate a lot of pain. Either way, you should not hesitate to contact your care team if you are experiencing pain. Talking about your pain is not "complaining" and ensuring your pain needs are met can improve quality of life.

Non-medicine treatments can also help with the stress and anxiety of having pain. Examples include massage, art or music therapy, acupuncture, relaxation, mindfulness (guided imagery), and cognitive behavior therapy (CBT). Radiation therapy can sometimes also help with pain, for example pain caused by bone metastases.

Sleep and wake issues

Sleep issues are common in those with cancer and cancer survivors. You might have trouble falling and staying asleep (insomnia). You might have difficulty staying awake during the day (somnolence). Side effects from cancer or its treatment might interrupt your sleep. You might have treatable conditions such as obstructive sleep apnea, restless legs syndrome, or periodic limb movement disorder. Your care team might change or add medicines or recommend a sleep study depending on your situation. Resting and getting enough sleep are important. Talk to your care team if your sleep or wake patterns has changed.

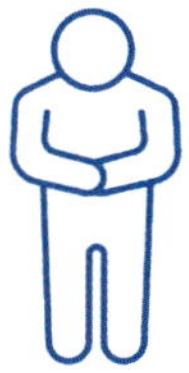

You know your body better than anyone

Help your care team understand:

- ✓ How you feel
- ✓ What you need
- ✓ What is working and what is not

Keep a list of names and contact information for each member of your team. This will make it easier for you and anyone involved in your care to know whom to contact with questions or concerns.

Get to know your care team and help them get to know you.

Wounds

A wound is a break in the skin or other body tissues caused by injury, pressure, infection, surgery, or cancer. A malignant wound happens when cancer cells travel from inside the body to the skin. This damages the skin and the blood and lymph vessels that support the skin, causing cell death. There are many ways to treat wounds based on the type of wound and its cause. A wound care specialist might be useful in some cases.

Psychosocial and spiritual distress

A cancer diagnosis and treatment can cause psychosocial and spiritual distress. Psychosocial has to do with mental, emotional, and social aspects of life. Some of the psychosocial effects of cancer are changes in how a person thinks, as well as their feelings, moods, beliefs, ways of coping, and relationships with family, friends, and coworkers.

Distress is an unpleasant experience of a mental, physical, social, or spiritual nature. Distress can include anxiety, depression, and difficulty sleeping. It can affect the way you think, feel, or act. Distress is normal during cancer care, but it may make it harder to cope with cancer. There are many ways to treat psychosocial and spiritual distress, such as counseling, education, group support, and spiritual support. Ask your care team for more information.

For more information, see NCCN Guidelines for Patients: Distress During Cancer Care, available at NCCN.org/patientguidelines and on the NCCN Patient Guides for Cancer app.

Mental health conditions

Some conditions that affect how we think, feel, and act need to be treated by a specialist such as a psychiatrist. A psychiatrist is a medical doctor who diagnoses and treats mental, emotional, and behavioral disorders.

Emotional and spiritual support

Psychologists, social workers, and spiritual care advisors such as hospital chaplains, personal clergy, or community representatives may provide help with easing distress.

Chaplains may be found in hospitals, mental health facilities, correctional institutions, children's hospitals, hospice centers, and nursing homes. They work with individuals, couples, families, and small groups, offering support and encouragement by:

- Listening to your concerns and offering comfort
- Answering ethical, moral, or religious questions
- Praying with you
- Providing rituals or sacraments
- Providing religious support and materials
- Offering end-of-life (EOL) emotional support
- Offering grief and bereavement counseling

Chaplains support and encourage people of all religious faiths and are familiar with beliefs across many different cultures. They often customize their approach based on an individual's background, age, or medical condition.

Social support and services

There are services to help with social and practical challenges or concerns. You may have concerns about:

- Family
- Money
- Getting to and from appointments (transportation)
- Safety
- Employment or loss of employment
- Access to food or housing
- Paying for health care, medicines, food, housing, or other expenses
- Taking care of yourself or others

Share any concerns you have with your care team.

Support from others

Family, friends, and coworkers can find it difficult to know how and when to support a person who has or had cancer. Reach out to others when you need help. Healing and recovery from the experience will take time. Everyone is different. Be clear whether you want to celebrate a milestone or anniversary. It's okay to change your mind!

Stress and coping

Coping skills are strategies a person uses to deal with stressful situations. These skills can be learned, and each person has a different way of coping. Eating a balanced diet, exercise, quality sleep, and fun or relaxing activities can help. Reach out for support to manage stress and build coping strategies.

Just as each person's cancer treatment is different, so are the ways of dealing with cancer.

- Practice ways to relax.
- Share your feelings with family, friends, a spiritual adviser, or a counselor.
- Keep a journal to help organize your thoughts.
- When faced with a difficult decision, list the pros and cons for each choice.
- Find a source of spiritual support.
- Set aside time to be alone.
- Remain involved with work and leisure activities as much as you can.
- Be ready to say no. This is the time to focus on you.

Grief and bereavement

Grief is deep sorrow or sadness caused by loss, such as the death of a friend or family member. Grief might also be felt by the person with cancer. Grief is a normal response to loss. Hospice and palliative care teams have expertise in how to provide support during this period.

- **Anticipatory grief or anticipatory mourning** is grief experienced by the person with cancer and their family and caregivers before death. It includes feelings of loss, concern for the dying person, balancing conflicting demands, and preparing for death.
- **Bereavement** is the period of sadness (grief) experienced by family and caregivers following a death. There is no right or wrong way to grieve. The process takes time.
- **Complicated grief** happens when grief does not progress as expected. When grief persists over a long period of time, it is important to seek help from a qualified professional. Complicated grief will not go away on its own.
- **Grief counseling** is used to help people cope with grief. Many hospice programs offer grief support, or they can refer you to another professional for help.

Bereavement care is often best provided by an experienced hospice team or a skilled mental health care professional. A well-supported end-of-life care experience can help with acceptance and bereavement.

"Don't let yourself stop doing the things you enjoy doing. Whatever your hobbies are, whatever things you like to do, keep doing them. It'll help you feel more like yourself and stay positive during what is an exhausting and mentally straining time."

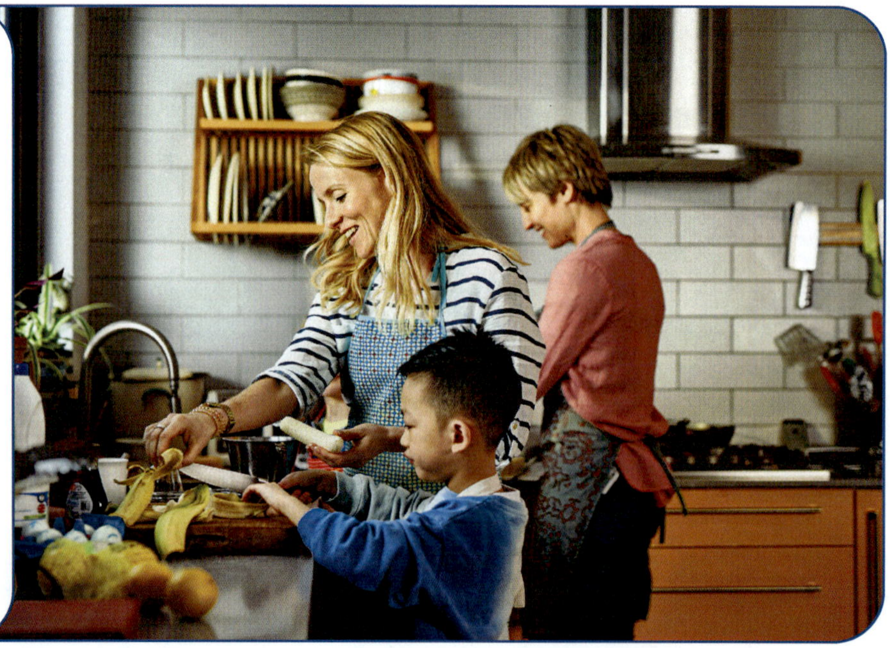

Key points

- A sign can be seen by someone else like your health care provider (HCP). A symptom is something only you can feel.
- Physical symptoms cause distress. Controlling symptoms and managing pain are an important part of cancer care.
- Pain and difficulty breathing are common physical symptoms experienced by those with cancer.
- A cancer diagnosis and treatment can cause psychosocial and spiritual distress. Psychosocial distress has to do with mental, emotional, and social aspects of life.
- Coping skills are strategies a person uses to deal with stressful situations. These skills can be learned, and each person has a different way of coping.
- Reach out to others, including your care team, when you need support.

Keep these things in mind

- Take care of yourself. This is a stressful time. Seek out and ask for support. Support can be a friend, relative, neighbor, or coworker.
- This will be a confusing time. You will hear a lot of unfamiliar words. Interact with your health care team, ask questions, and talk about how you feel.

3
Communicating with your care team

19 Communication is key

19 About cancer treatment

20 Advance directives

21 MOLST or POLST

21 Life-sustaining treatments

22 Key points

Shared decision-making is an important part of person-centered cancer care, including palliative care and advance care planning. In shared decision-making, you and your care team discuss and weigh options, and decide on a care plan that is right for you.

Communication is key

Shared decision-making (SDM) is an important part of person-centered cancer care, including palliative care and advance care planning. Together, you and your care team will discuss and weigh options, and decide on a care plan. Most people want to be involved in decisions about their health care. When people are involved in decisions about their care, they experience a greater sense of control, higher satisfaction, and improved quality of life.

We don't always know what questions to ask or how to start the conversation about what we want from a care plan. This book may give you some ideas of questions to ask at your next visit. Some people find it helpful to write questions down in advance and bring them to their appointment. It may be helpful to have a friend or family member attend appointments with you to take notes or ask their own questions. It is also okay if you don't have any questions.

About cancer treatment

Cancer treatment will be based on your preferences and goals of treatment, and the features of your tumor, cancer, or cancer status. Many factors play a role in how the cancer responds to treatment. It is important to have regular talks with your care team about how treatment is working for you, including how it is impacting your ability to live your life the way you want.

For specific treatment recommendations about your type of cancer, see the complete list of NCCN Guidelines for Patients at NCCN.org/patientguidelines and on the NCCN Patient Guides for Cancer app.

What is a prognosis?

When a person and their family first learn of a cancer diagnosis, they often want to know what this means for them. A prognosis is a way that your cancer team tries to answer the question about what this cancer means for your care plan, how you'll live your life, and how long you'll live your life. Prognostic awareness (PA) is a person's knowledge and understanding of the course their life is likely to take. A prognosis can change in response to treatment. For example, if a treatment can control your cancer, you might live longer if you receive that treatment. Consider if you want your doctor to talk about your prognosis.

Shared decision-making and advance care planning

When facing a cancer diagnosis, it may be a good time to share with family and friends how you feel about life, your body, and your hopes and worries. Discussing the future in this way is called advance care planning. Thinking about what is important to you can help with shared decision-making now and in the future.

Help your care team understand what matters to you and how this influences your views about cancer treatments and quality of life. Discuss the benefits and burdens of medicines or therapies that are recommended and how they might impact your quality of life in both positive and negative ways. Include family, friends, and caregivers in these conversations, as needed.

It is also important for everyone, especially if you are receiving medical care, to have a health care proxy. A health care proxy (also called the durable power of attorney for health care or DPAHC) allows you to choose someone to make medical decisions for you if you ever became unable to speak for yourself. When you choose a health care proxy, it is important to talk to the person you choose about the things that you do or don't want.

If your cancer team and health care proxy understand what is most important to you, it can help ensure that you always receive the care that you would want, even if something were to happen and you were unable to speak for yourself.

Advance directives

Advance directives (ADs) are only a part of the larger care planning conversation. Advance directives are legal documents in which you write out ahead of time what types of medical care you would want if you ever became unable to speak for yourself. They include naming a health care agent who would make decisions if you were unable to tell the doctors yourself. Most advance directives include a living will section that allows you to provide information about your goals and values that may inform future decision-making, including at the end of life (EOL). Some advance directives will ask about preferences for specific treatments such as breathing tubes, CPR (cardiopulmonary resuscitation), dialysis, or tube feeding. Advance directives do not expire, but you can change or revoke an advance directive at any time.

How do I choose a health care agent or proxy?

Name the person who will make health care decisions for you (health care proxy, agent, or surrogate) in the advance directive. This person may have to make some very tough decisions. Choose carefully when selecting your proxy and make sure the proxy feels comfortable representing you.

Think about someone who:

- You know and trust
- Can separate their own wishes from yours
- You know would carry out your wishes
- Could be easily reached
- Could handle it if other family members or loved ones wanted you to get treated differently than you would want

Some people choose a second person as an alternate proxy, in case their first choice cannot be reached at the time decisions need to be made.

MOLST or POLST

Medical Orders for Life-Sustaining Treatment (MOLST) or Physician Orders for Life-Sustaining Treatment (POLST) is a type of advance directive that you may complete with your doctor. It is signed by both of you. These forms are not available in every state and are often used when someone has a clear preference, such as to avoid CPR. If MOLST or POLST isn't available in your state, there may be another order that your doctor can write to ensure your wishes are respected.

Life-sustaining treatments

Life-sustaining or life-prolonging treatments attempt to extend life and can include the use of machines. This equipment does the work for an organ, such as:

- A machine to help with breathing (ventilator)
- A machine to help your kidneys (dialysis)
- A tube placed into your stomach to provide food, nutrition, and medicines (nasogastric or gastrostomy tube)
- A tube placed into your vein to provide fluids and medicines (intravenous, IV tube)
- A tube or mask used to supply oxygen

Sometimes life-sustaining treatments are temporary to help your medical condition improve and sometimes they are used for a longer time. It is helpful to think about what is most important to you and situations where life-sustaining treatments may or may not be within your goals of care. Each person's definition of what makes life worth living is unique and will influence these kinds of decisions. We may not know what will happen in the future, but sharing what matters most with your cancer team, family, and friends will help to ensure the right care plan for you.

Hospice and end-of-life care

People who are approaching the end of life (EOL) often find that cancer-directed treatments and life-sustaining treatments have more burdens than benefits. For people with a life expectancy of 6 months or less who decide to shift their focus towards comfort at the end of life, hospice is a service that can provide a special kind of EOL care. Hospice care is specifically designed for individuals with a limited life expectancy. It focuses on providing comfort and support to people and their families by providing care providers and resources that specialize in EOL care. Hospice care can be at home or at an inpatient center. It can also include respite care. Respite care provides short-term relief for caregivers. If you have questions about hospice, bring them up with your care team.

Key points

- Shared decision-making (SDM) is an important part of person-centered cancer care. When people are involved in decisions about their care, they experience a greater sense of control, higher satisfaction, and improved quality of life.
- Cancer treatment should be based on your individual needs, type of cancer, and your preferences and goals.
- Advance care planning (ACP) includes making decisions now about the care you would want to receive if you became unable to speak for yourself. Advance care planning is for everyone.
- Advance directives (ADs) are legal documents in which you write out ahead of time what types of medical care you would want if you ever became unable to speak for yourself. They include naming a health care agent.
- A health care proxy (also called the durable power of attorney for health care or DPAHC) allows you to choose someone to make medical decisions for you if you ever became unable to speak for yourself.
- Hospice care is specifically designed for individuals with a limited life expectancy. It focuses on providing comfort and support to people and their families by providing care providers and resources that specialize in end-of-life care.

> “Be your own advocate. Talk to someone who has gone through the same thing as you. Ask important questions, even the ones you are afraid to ask. You have to protect yourself and ensure you make the best decisions for you, and get the best care for your particular situation.”

5

Making treatment decisions

24 It's your choice

24 Questions to ask

32 Resources

It's important to be comfortable with the cancer treatment you choose. This choice starts with having an open and honest conversation with your care team.

It's your choice

In shared decision-making, you and your care team share information, discuss the options, and agree on a treatment plan. It starts with an open and honest conversation between you and your care team.

Treatment decisions are very personal. What is important to you may not be important to someone else.

Some things that may play a role in your decision-making:

- What you want and how that might differ from what others want
- Your religious and spiritual beliefs
- Your feelings about certain treatments
- Your feelings about pain or side effects
- Cost of treatment, travel to treatment centers, and time away from school or work
- Quality of life and length of life
- How active you are and the activities that are important to you

Think about what you want from treatment. Discuss openly the risks and benefits of specific treatments and procedures. Weigh options and share concerns with your care team. If you take the time to build a relationship with your care team, it will help you feel supported when considering options and making treatment decisions.

Second opinion

It is normal to want to start treatment as soon as possible. While cancer can't be ignored, there is time to have another doctor review your test results and suggest a treatment plan. This is called getting a second opinion, and it's a normal part of cancer care. Even doctors get second opinions!

Things you can do to prepare:

- Check with your insurance company about its rules on second opinions. There may be out-of-pocket costs to see doctors who are not part of your insurance plan.
- Make plans to have copies of all your records sent to the doctor you will see for your second opinion.

Support groups

Many people diagnosed with cancer find support groups to be helpful. Support groups often include people at different stages of treatment. Some people may be newly diagnosed, while others may be finished with treatment. If your hospital or community doesn't have support groups for people with cancer, check out the websites listed in this book.

Questions to ask

Possible questions to ask your care team are listed on the following pages. Feel free to use these questions or come up with your own.

Questions about your care team's experience

1. What is your experience treating this cancer? What else do you treat?
2. What is the experience of those on your team?
3. How many people like me (of the same age, gender, race) have you treated?
4. Will you be consulting with experts to discuss my care? Whom will you consult?
5. How many procedures like the one you're suggesting have you done?
6. Is this treatment a major part of your practice?
7. How many of your patients have had complications? What were the complications?
8. Who will manage my day-to-day care?

Questions about options

1. What will happen if I do nothing?
2. How do my age, overall health, and other factors affect the options?
3. Which option is proven to work best for my cancer, age, overall health, and other factors?
4. What are the possible complications and side effects? Are any life-threatening?
5. What can be done to prevent or relieve the side effects of treatment?
6. Am I a candidate for a clinical trial? Can I join a clinical trial at any time?
7. What decisions must be made today?
8. Is there a social worker or someone who can help me decide about treatment?
9. Is there a hospital or treatment center you can recommend for treatment?
10. Can I go to one hospital for surgery and a different center for radiation therapy?

Questions about treatment

1. Which treatment(s) do you recommend and why?
2. Does the order of treatment matter?
3. When will I start treatment?
4. How long will treatment likely take?
5. What should I expect from treatment?
6. What will you do to make me comfortable during treatment?
7. What are the chances my cancer will return after treatment?
8. I would like a second opinion. Is there someone you can recommend?

Questions about side effects

1. What are the side effects of this treatment?
2. How are these side effects treated?
3. How long will these side effects last?
4. What side effects should I watch for that could be life-threatening?
5. When should I call my care team?
6. What should I do on weekends and other non-office hours?
7. What emergency department or ER should I go to?
8. Will my treatment team be able to communicate with the ER team?
9. What medicines can I take to prevent or relieve side effects?
10. What can I do to help with pain and other side effects?

Questions about resources and support

1. Who can I talk to about help with housing, food, and other basic needs?
2. What help is available for transportation, childcare, and home care?
3. How much will I have to pay for treatment?
4. Who can tell me about health insurance options and help me apply for insurance coverage?
5. What help is available to pay for medicines and other treatment?
6. What other services are available to me and my caregivers?
7. How can I connect with others and build a support system?
8. How can I find in-person or online support?
9. Who can help me with my concerns about missing work or school?
10. Who can I talk to if I don't feel safe at home, at work, or in my neighborhood?

Questions about end-of-life care

1. What can I expect as my cancer progresses?
2. How will I feel?
3. What symptoms will I have and how will they be treated?
4. Will I be able to think clearly and get out of bed?
5. What happens during end-of-life (EOL) care?
6. What decisions need to be made to prepare for and during EOL care?
7. How much will this treatment extend my life?
8. How much time will I spend traveling to and from appointments and having treatment?
9. Does this hospital have an EOL support program for people my age? Please refer me to a counselor or support group who can help me and my family.

Questions about hospice care

1. When does hospice care start?
2. Who decides when it is time to enter hospice care?
3. Who will help arrange for hospice care?
4. What will be done to manage my pain and other symptoms?
5. What medicines or treatments should stop? When?
6. How can I find out if hospice is covered by my insurance?
7. Where will my hospice care take place?
8. Is there a chance I will be in and out of hospice care?

Resources

Breastcancer.org
Breastcancer.org

Breast Cancer Alliance
breastcanceralliance.org

DiepC Foundation
DiepCfoundation.org

FORCE: Facing Our Risk of Cancer Empowered
facingourrisk.org

MedlinePlus
medlineplus.gov

National Cancer Institute (NCI)
cancer.gov

National Institute on Aging
nia.nih.gov

Ovarcome
Ovarcome.org

Ovarian Cancer Research Alliance
ocrahope.org

Sharsheret
sharsheret.org

The Leukemia & Lymphoma Society
LLS.org/PatientSupport

Triage Cancer
triagecancer.org

Unite for HER
Uniteforher.org

World Health Organization (WHO)
who.int/health-topics/palliative-care

share with us.

**Take our survey,
and help make the
NCCN Guidelines for Patients
better for everyone!**

NCCN.org/patients/comments

Words to know

advance care planning (ACP)
Making decisions now about the care you would want to receive if you became unable to speak for yourself.

advance directive (AD)
Legal document in which you write out ahead of time what types of medical care you would want if you ever became unable to speak for yourself. There is more than one type of advance directive.

anxiety
A feeling of fear, dread, and uneasiness.

bereavement
Period of time grief is experienced after a death.

delirium
A mental state in which a person is confused and has reduced awareness of their surroundings. Delirium can also cause hallucinations. Delirium may be caused by infection, dehydration, abnormal levels of some electrolytes, organ failure, medicines, or serious illness, such as advanced cancer.

depression
A mood disorder that causes a persistent feeling of sadness and loss of interest in daily activities.

distress
Extreme anxiety, sorrow, or pain.

end-of-life (EOL) care
Care given to people who are near the end of life and have stopped treatment to cure or control their disease. End-of-life care may include hospice care. Also called comfort care.

grief
Deep sorrow or sadness caused by loss, such as the death of a friend or family member. Grief might also be felt by the person with cancer.

health care proxy
A type of advance directive that gives a person (such as a relative, lawyer, or friend) the authority to make health care decisions for another person. It becomes active when that person loses the ability to make decisions. Also called health care agent or surrogate.

hospice care
A program that gives special care to people who are near the end of life and have stopped treatment to cure or control their disease.

life-sustaining or life-extending treatment
Treatment that extends life such as cardiopulmonary resuscitation (CPR) and fluid resuscitation. Includes the use of machines.

Medical Orders for Life-Sustaining Treatment (MOLST) or Physician Orders for Life-Sustaining Treatment (POLST)
A form that documents a person's preferences for life-sustaining treatments such as cardiopulmonary resuscitation (CPR). It is signed by a person and their doctor and is part of the medical record.

palliative
Reduces the severity of a disease or symptom without curing it.

palliative care
Specialized care given to improve quality of life and help reduce physical, mental, emotional, and spiritual distress.

palliative care specialist
A health care professional who is specifically trained in palliative care to provide in-depth pain and symptom management, communication regarding goals of care, and care coordination across settings and over time.

prognosis
The likely course and outcome of a disease.

prognostic awareness (PA)
A person's knowledge and understanding of the course their disease is likely to take.

psychosocial
Having to do with the mental, emotional, social, and spiritual aspects.

psychosocial support
Support given to help meet mental, emotional, and social needs.

quality of life (QOL)
General well-being.

side effect
An unhealthy or unpleasant physical or emotional response to treatment.

sign
Can be seen or measured by someone else.

spiritual
Having to do with religious beliefs.

symptom
Something only you can feel such as pain or nausea.

We want your feedback!

Our goal is to provide helpful and easy-to-understand information on cancer.

Take our survey to let us know what we got right and what we could do better.

NCCN.org/patients/feedback

NCCN Contributors

This patient guide is based on the NCCN Clinical Practice Guidelines in Oncology (NCCN Guidelines®) for Palliative Care Version 2.2023. It was adapted, reviewed, and published with help from the following people:

Dorothy A. Shead, MS
Senior Director
Patient Information Operations

Tanya Fischer, MEd, MSLIS
Senior Medical Writer, Patient Information

Laura Phillips
Graphic Artist

The NCCN Clinical Practice Guidelines in Oncology (NCCN Guidelines®) for Palliative Care Version 2.2023 were developed by the following NCCN Panel Members:

Maria Dans, MD/Chair
Siteman Cancer Center at Barnes-Jewish Hospital and Washington University School of Medicine

*Anne M. Walling, MD, PhD/Vice-Chair
UCLA Jonsson Comprehensive Cancer Center

Rajiv Agarwal, MD
Vanderbilt-Ingram Cancer Center

Jessica R. Bauman, MD
Fox Chase Cancer Center

Anna C. Beck, MD
Huntsman Cancer Institute at the University of Utah

*Toby C. Campbell, MD, MSCI
University of Wisconsin Carbone Cancer Center

*Elise C. Carey, MD
Mayo Clinic Comprehensive Cancer Center

Amy A. Case, MD
Roswell Park Comprehensive Cancer Center

Shalini Dalal, MD
The University of Texas MD Anderson Cancer Center

Danielle J. Doberman, MD, MPH
The Sidney Kimmel Comprehensive Cancer Center at Johns Hopkins

Andrew S. Epstein, MD
Memorial Sloan Kettering Cancer Center

*Nathan Paul Fairman, MD, MPH
UC Davis Comprehensive Cancer Center

Leslie Fecher, MD
University of Michigan Rogel Cancer Center

Stacy Fischer, MD
University of Colorado Cancer Center

Joshua Jones, MD, MA
Abramson Cancer Center at the University of Pennsylvania

Jennifer Kapo, MD
Yale Cancer Center/Smilow Cancer Hospital

Deena Levine, MD
St. Jude Children's Research Hospital/ The University of Tennessee Health Science Center

Elizabeth T. Loggers, MD, PhD
Fred Hutchinson Cancer Center

Susan McCammon, MD
O'Neal Comprehensive Cancer Center at UAB

Erin Newton, MD
Indiana University Melvin and Bren Simon Comprehensive Cancer Center

*Adeboye B. Ogunseitan, MD
Robert H. Lurie Comprehensive Cancer Center of Northwestern University

*Sahana Rajasekhara, MD
Moffitt Cancer Center

Kavitha Ramchandran, MD
Stanford Cancer Institute

Kira Skavinski, DO
UC San Diego Moores Cancer Center

Linda Sutton, MD
Duke Cancer Institute

Jennifer Temel, MD
Massachusetts General Hospital Cancer Center

Melissa L. Teply, MD
Fred & Pamela Buffett Cancer Center

Stephanie Y. Terauchi, MD
UT Southwestern Simmons Comprehensive Cancer Center

Jane Thomas, MD
Dana-Farber/Brigham and Women's Cancer Center

Sharla Wells-Di-Gregorio, PhD
The Ohio State University Comprehensive Cancer Center - James Cancer Hospital and Solove Research Institute

*Finly Zachariah, MD
City of Hope National Medical Center

Nicholas G. Zaorsky, MD, MS
Case Comprehensive Cancer Center/ University Hospitals Seidman Cancer Center and Cleveland Clinic Taussig Cancer Institute

NCCN

Carly J. Cassara, MSc
Guidelines Layout Specialist

Kevin Pang, PharmD
Associate Scientist/Medical Writer

* Reviewed this patient guide. For disclosures, visit NCCN.org/disclosures.

NCCN Cancer Centers

Abramson Cancer Center
at the University of Pennsylvania
Philadelphia, Pennsylvania
800.789.7366 • pennmedicine.org/cancer

Case Comprehensive Cancer Center/
University Hospitals Seidman Cancer Center and
Cleveland Clinic Taussig Cancer Institute
Cleveland, Ohio
UH Seidman Cancer Center
800.641.2422 • uhhospitals.org/services/cancer-services
CC Taussig Cancer Institute
866.223.8100 • my.clevelandclinic.org/departments/cancer
Case CCC
216.844.8797 • case.edu/cancer

City of Hope National Medical Center
Duarte, California
800.826.4673 • cityofhope.org

Dana-Farber/Brigham and Women's Cancer Center |
Mass General Cancer Center
Boston, Massachusetts
617.732.5500 • youhaveus.org
617.726.5130 • massgeneral.org/cancer-center

Duke Cancer Institute
Durham, North Carolina
888.275.3853 • dukecancerinstitute.org

Fox Chase Cancer Center
Philadelphia, Pennsylvania
888.369.2427 • foxchase.org

Fred & Pamela Buffett Cancer Center
Omaha, Nebraska
402.559.5600 • unmc.edu/cancercenter

Fred Hutchinson Cancer Center
Seattle, Washington
206.667.5000 • fredhutch.org

Huntsman Cancer Institute at the University of Utah
Salt Lake City, Utah
800.824.2073 • healthcare.utah.edu/huntsmancancerinstitute

Indiana University Melvin and Bren Simon
Comprehensive Cancer Center
Indianapolis, Indiana
888.600.4822 • www.cancer.iu.edu

Mayo Clinic Comprehensive Cancer Center
Phoenix/Scottsdale, Arizona
Jacksonville, Florida
Rochester, Minnesota
480.301.8000 • Arizona
904.953.0853 • Florida
507.538.3270 • Minnesota
mayoclinic.org/cancercenter

Memorial Sloan Kettering Cancer Center
New York, New York
800.525.2225 • mskcc.org

Moffitt Cancer Center
Tampa, Florida
888.663.3488 • moffitt.org

O'Neal Comprehensive Cancer Center at UAB
Birmingham, Alabama
800.822.0933 • uab.edu/onealcancercenter

Robert H. Lurie Comprehensive Cancer Center
of Northwestern University
Chicago, Illinois
866.587.4322 • cancer.northwestern.edu

Roswell Park Comprehensive Cancer Center
Buffalo, New York
877.275.7724 • roswellpark.org

Siteman Cancer Center at Barnes-Jewish Hospital
and Washington University School of Medicine
St. Louis, Missouri
800.600.3606 • siteman.wustl.edu

St. Jude Children's Research Hospital/
The University of Tennessee Health Science Center
Memphis, Tennessee
866.278.5833 • stjude.org
901.448.5500 • uthsc.edu

Stanford Cancer Institute
Stanford, California
877.668.7535 • cancer.stanford.edu

The Ohio State University Comprehensive Cancer Center -
James Cancer Hospital and Solove Research Institute
Columbus, Ohio
800.293.5066 • cancer.osu.edu

The Sidney Kimmel Comprehensive
Cancer Center at Johns Hopkins
Baltimore, Maryland
410.955.8964
www.hopkinskimmelcancercenter.org

The UChicago Medicine Comprehensive Cancer Center
Chicago, Illinois
773.702.1000 • uchicagomedicine.org/cancer

The University of Texas MD Anderson Cancer Center
Houston, Texas
844.269.5922 • mdanderson.org

UC Davis Comprehensive Cancer Center
Sacramento, California
916.734.5959 • 800.770.9261
health.ucdavis.edu/cancer

UC San Diego Moores Cancer Center
La Jolla, California
858.822.6100 • cancer.ucsd.edu

UCLA Jonsson Comprehensive Cancer Center
Los Angeles, California
310.825.5268 • cancer.ucla.edu

UCSF Helen Diller Family
Comprehensive Cancer Center
San Francisco, California
800.689.8273 • cancer.ucsf.edu

University of Colorado Cancer Center
Aurora, Colorado
720.848.0300 • coloradocancercenter.org

University of Michigan Rogel Cancer Center
Ann Arbor, Michigan
800.865.1125 • rogelcancercenter.org

University of Wisconsin Carbone Cancer Center
Madison, Wisconsin
608.265.1700 • uwhealth.org/cancer

UT Southwestern Simmons
Comprehensive Cancer Center
Dallas, Texas
214.648.3111 • utsouthwestern.edu/simmons

Vanderbilt-Ingram Cancer Center
Nashville, Tennessee
877.936.8422 • vicc.org

Yale Cancer Center/Smilow Cancer Hospital
New Haven, Connecticut
855.4.SMILOW • yalecancercenter.org

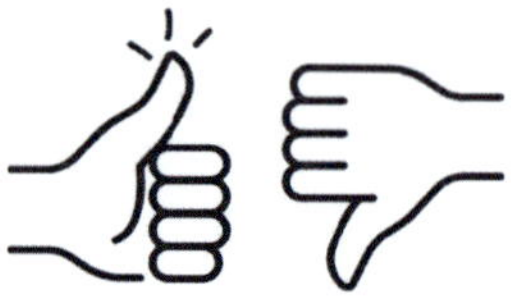

Let us know what you think!

Please take a moment to complete an online survey about the NCCN Guidelines for Patients.

NCCN.org/patients/response

Notes

Index

advance care planning (ACP) 21

advance directive (AD) 20–21

cancer treatment 19

care team 5–7

constipation 10

delirium 10–11

diarrhea 11

difficulty breathing 11

distress 14

emotional distress 14–16

end-of-life (EOL) care 21

fatigue 12

grief 16

health care proxy 20

hospice care 6, 21

life-sustaining treatment 21

loss of appetite 12

lymphedema 12

mental health conditions 14

nausea and vomiting 12

pain 13

palliative care specialists 7

physical symptoms 10–13

shared decision-making (SDM) 19–20, 24

sleep and wake issues 13

social support 15

spiritual distress 14–16

spiritual support 14

weight loss 12

wounds 13

Made in United States
North Haven, CT
11 November 2023

43887604R00024